The Instant Pot

A Guide To Cooking Delicious Dishes

Marcus S. Dowd

Contents

Chapter One

Introduction

The Instant Pot is an electric pressure cooker that cooks food quickly

Cooking Delectable Dishes: A Guide

Author

Marcus S. Dowd

It comes with a pressure setting, a built-in warming component, and several cooking modules that make cooking as simple as possible. Food that is robotized and low-cost is being developed by Moment Pot. An Instant Pot's design includes a pre-programmed electric warming source as well as a timer to manage the cooking time. You can cook almost anything using the Instant Pot's basic kitchen setting. You may prepare healthful morning meals in a couple of minutes, satisfy your voracious hunger with go-to snacks, or pamper your sweet taste with mouth-watering desserts with this cutting-edge equipment.

With a versatile Instant Pot, you may prepare stew, soup, stew, beans, different types of meat, lentils, veggies, oatmeal, and more. It may be used as a standard cooking machine for sautéing, stewing, or simple preheating. An Instant Pot is a multi-functional kitchen appliance that may be used as a slow cooker, rice cooker, or yogurt maker.

You'll get a limited selection of 100 Instant Pot ideas to prepare various cuisines at the comfort of your own home in this fantastic Instant Pot cookbook. Morning meals, canapés, sides, grains, rice, soups, stews, main course, snacks, stocks, sauces, pastries, and yogurts, as well as main course dinners, are now available to prepare from your favorite ingredients. This book has a number of veggie-friendly dinners, as well as main-course meals made with chicken, red meat, and fish.

Don't be a bystander; let's start by executing some of your most treasured goals and investigating a novel approach of preparing foods. Chapter 2: Instant Pot's Wonderful World

The Instant Pot is an excellent investment and a valuable kitchen tool. You may also cook food in large batches, freeze it, and then reheat it later.

It's never been easier to prepare your favorite cuisines. All you have to do now is toss everything into the pot and call it a day. It makes use of limited steam to let you make delectable feasts in record time. The majority of supplements in meals may be fixed with the use of Moment Pot.

Chapter Two

WHY IS IT CALLED A KITCHEN REVOLUTION ABOVE AND BEYOND THE BASICS?

Time and energy are both saved.

When compared to other cooking methods, the Instant Pot invests in some possibility to plan meals. Dry fixings such as beans, grains, veggies, and heartbeats work marvelously in this machine. You may just add them to the pot, along with the recommended amount of fluids and other ingredients, instead of pre-soaking them for 2 to 12 hours ahead to cooking time. You may cook them in less than 30 minutes at high strain.

Microorganisms are extinguished.

The water level is heated to a high degree in the Instant Pot, killing the bulk of the unwanted microscopic critters. It eliminates harmful bacteria and parasites from grains and vegetables, ensuring that you always have a delicious meal.

Diet and Fitness

Unlike many other cooking methods, which need you to submerge the veggies and other ingredients entirely in water to cook them, the moment pot just requires a little amount of water to maintain high steam levels. This technique prevents the erosion of essential components.

Effortless Cooking

Poultry, soup, rice, beans/stew, meat/stew, porridges, multi-grain, steam, and other control keys are all included in an Instant Pot's 12-key capacity. Every mode offers pressure and timing settings that you may alter to suit your needs.

Buttons for the Instant Pot, third chapter

With a variety of pre-programmed cooking modules, the Instant Pot gives you the most up-to-date culinary capabilities and can prepare anything for you. The following are typical cooking settings.

This option is for browning, sautéing, or simmering of additional ingredients such as oil, garlic, onions, and other vegetables with the lid open.

Slow Cook Button: This feature transforms your Instant Pot into a rice cooker, capable of cooking for up to 40 hours, however the normal setting is 4 hours.

Soup Button: This option allows you to make a variety of broths and soups quickly and effortlessly. 30 to 35 minutes of high pressure is the default setting.

The default setting for the Poultry Button is high pressure for 18 to 20 minutes.

Porridge Button: This option makes it simple to make oatmeal or porridge with a variety of grains. High pressure for 20 to 25 minutes is the default setting.

You may manually set your own pressure and cook time using the Manual Button.

Button for Beans/Chili: This option allows you to quickly make chili or beans. For 30 to 35 minutes, the default setting is high pressure.

Meat/Stew Button: This setting makes it simple to cook meats or stews, and it's set to high pressure for 35 to 40 minutes by default.

Keep Warm/Cancel Button: This feature allows you to cancel any previously run program, as well as put the cooker on standby and keep it warm for a period of time.

Rice Button: Your Instant Pot becomes a rice cooker when you use this feature. You can easily make a variety of rice-based dishes and other cuisines with this setting. The automated option for this setting cooks rice at low pressure and is the default. To choose your preferred time, utilize the "Adjust" option.

Cake & Egg Button: This option allows you to prepare a variety of cake and egg-based dishes.

Multigrain Button: This option allows you to quickly make a variety of grains, such as beans, brown rice, and wild rice. This setting's default is for 40 to 45 minutes of high intensity.

pressure. Use the Steam Button to steam seafood, vegetables, or reheat meals. Normally, high-pressure cooking takes 10 to 15 minutes.

The default option for the Yogurt Button is 8 hours of cooking time for various types of yogurt. You may also use "Change" to increase or decrease the amount of time you spend on the computer.

How Does It Work?, Chapter 4

The Instant Pot differs from a traditional strain cooker in that it has several settings that allow you to prepare a variety of foods. What is the purpose of this computerized pressure cooker? To understand how it works, you must first get acquainted with its components and many fasteners.

Features

The Instant Pot is an ingenious device that allows you to cook a large number of dishes in a short amount of time.

dishes prepared using a single device The Instant Pot has the following features that make it one of the best computerized pressure cookers on the market.

Many programmable settings: Depending on the option you choose on the Instant Pot, you may control the cooking time and temperature within the Instant Pot. Later in this part, we'll talk about the programmable settings.

Sleek appearance: The Instant Pot's sleek exterior not only makes cleaning a breeze, but it also lends sophistication to the overall kitchen appliance.

Delay cooking timer: The Instant Pot may be turned into a delayed cooker, allowing you to prepare meals later and have it ready when you return. Once you've returned home, you'll be able to eat warm, soothing meals.

People are hesitant to use the pressure cooker because they are skeptical of the device's safety features. The Instant Pot, on the other hand, contains a number of safety safeguards to ensure that the gadget functions correctly and does not overheat. It contains a pressure sensor that detects excessive pressure within the pot and shuts it off immediately.

it is released It also features an internal regulator that allows you to monitor the precise temperature at which your food is cooking. Finally, the quick tension delivery allows you to rapidly ease the strain in the pot.

Other important accessories are included: The Instant Pot comes with a number of useful attachments to expand its capabilities. Silicone mittens, steamer rack, condensation collector, rice paddle, soup spoon, and measuring cup are among the useful accessories that come with your Instant Pot.

Cleaning Hints, Chapter 5

To keep up with the Instant Pot's display, it's important to clean it often. It is simply cleaning the Instant Pot. Indeed, there are so many incredible cleaning suggestions for the Instant Pot out there that we just listed the best cleaning methods to maintain your computerized pressure cooker in tip-top shape.

Separate the internal pot from the Instant Pot gently: Unlike other pressure cookers, only the inner pot of the Instant Pot becomes filthy. Remove the inside pot as soon as possible so that it may be thoroughly cleaned afterwards. To remove any hardened food particles from the outside body, dampen a clean towel with warm water softly. Also, never submerge the outside body in water since it houses all of the electrical components that allow the machine to function.

Now immediately disconnect the Instant Pot from the power source: Before cleaning the Instant Pot, ensure sure it is unplugged from the power supply to avoid electrocution. It's also a good idea to inspect the cable for any damage.

Allow for drying before reassembling the Instant Pot: Before reassembling the Instant Pot, allow all components to dry at room temperature. Please double-check that everything, particularly the electrical cables, are securely fastened before reassembling.

The only washable parts of the Instant Pot are the inside pot and the cover. After that, give them a short wash in warm, soapy water. The inner pot may be washed in the dishwasher as well. Before putting them back together in the Instant Pot, ensure sure they've dried completely.

Please clean the lid with care: The lid is made up of many components and should be handled with care. Remove the steam release handle first, and then inspect for any trapped food particles. Remove the silicone sealing ring and examine for damages and hardened food particles.

Finish with a dollop of whip cream and a scattering of chocolate shavings.

4 to 5 servings

5–10 minutes of preparation time 10–15 minutes of cooking time The huge formula that follows... Information about the calories:

Serving size: 173 calories 35.5 g carbs 6.4 gram of protein

5.1 gram fat 4 g fibre

Cornmeal Porridge with Coconut It's unquestionably a show-stealer.

Ingredients:

a quarter-cup coconut milk

3/4 cup thick milk, enhanced

1 14 cup finely ground yellow cornmeal

1 tsp. coconut flakes (about 1 teaspoon)

Cinnamon sticks, 2 1/2

1 1/4 tsp vanilla

6 oz.

Directions:

First and foremost, make sure you have all of the necessary fixings on hand. In the Instant Pot, combine 5 cups water and the whole can of coconut milk.

Combine the cornmeal and 1 cup of water in a blender, then pour the mixture into the saucepan.

This is a tremendous development. Vanilla extract, coconut drops, and cinnamon sticks are added to the mixture.

After that, close the cooker's lid and choose "Manual" as the work mode.

Cook at high pressure for 5 to 10 minutes, depending on the chance.

There is one more task to do. Release the tension normally and remove the lid after the signal has been received.

Finally, combine the enhanced consolidated milk with the rest of the ingredients.

6 to 7 servings

15 to 20 minutes of prep time

5–10 minutes of cooking time During tests, I used to create them. Information about the calories:

There are 253 calories in a single serving of this recipe. 46.2 grams of carbohydrate

6.9 g protien 3.1 gram fat 17.2g sugar

179mg sodium

Steel Cut Vanilla Oats are the ultimate in deliciousness. This is quite simple to create.

Ingredients:

•\s•\s•\s•\s•\s•\s•\s•\s•

1 pound oats, steel-cut

Serve with grated chocolate. Whipped cream for serving 2 and 1/2 cups water a pinch of salt and around 2.5 tablespoons sugar 2 tsp vanilla

1 tsp. de café 1 quart of cream

Directions:

To begin, double-check that you have all of the necessary supplies. In your current pot, combine the oats, milk, water, sugar, salt, and coffee powder; stir well, cover, and cook on High for 10 to 15 minutes. Cook on High for 10 minutes with the lid on.

Finally, stir in the vanilla concentrate, let aside for 5 to 10 minutes, then divide amongst dishes and top with whipped cream and crushed chocolate. Enjoy!

10 to 15 minutes for preparation 10–15 minutes of cooking time 4–5 portions Get set, get set, get set, get set, get set, get set, get

Information about the calories:

250 calories, 3.1 grams of fat, 5.4 grams of fiber

Iconic Scotch Eggs With Ground Sausage (43 g carbs, 4 g sugar, 5 g protein)

Some are a little out of the norm, while others are a little unusual. Ingredients:

•\s•\s•\s•\s•\s•

1. 2. 3. 4. 5. 6. 7. 8. 9. 10. Directions: 1. 2. 3. 4.

1 pound of sausage (ground)

1/2 tsp mint (dried) Vegetable oil (about 1.5 tbsp.) 1 tsp cayenne 1 salt pinch

Eggs, 4

To begin, double-check that you have all of the necessary fixings. In your Instant Pot, put the steaming bin in. Add 1 cup of water to the eggs at this time.

Close the lid of your Instant Pot and set the timer for 5 to 10 minutes on high pressure.

When the timer goes off, let the strain out for 5 to 10 minutes, then use the Instant Pot for a quick delivery and mood boost.

This is a tremendous development. After cooling the eggs in cold water, remove the shells and cut the hotdog into equal-sized pieces.

Then, using your fingers, season the frankfurter with salt, pepper, and mint. Flatten the wiener meat into equal-sized pieces, then place your hard-boiled eggs in the center, folding your frankfurter over it.

Re-enact the process with the remaining egg halves. In your Instant Pot, press the sauté or cooking option and add a little amount of oil (no more than 3 tablespoons) to sauté your scotch eggs.

Remove the eggs from the Instant Pot and fill it with 1 cup of water after the sautéing has completed.

There is one more task to do. Place the trivet on top of the rack or trivet and place the eggs on top of the eggs. Finally, set the tension to high for 5 to 10 minutes, then quickly release the strain and serve your scotch rolls when the timer goes off. Enjoy! 15- to 20-minute time frame

4–6 people Overcoming the adversity...

Information about the calories: Cholesterol 0mg Calories 280g Fats 18.7g

Carbohydrates in their Total Form 12g protein, 16g carbohydrates

Casserole de Ham et d'Oeuf The most amazing recipe I've ever encountered.

Ingredients:

•\s•\s•\s•\s•\s•

ham, 1 cup (Diced)

1 teaspoon pepper, dark chives (1/4 cup) (Chopped)

1 cup Greek yogurt, plain 6 eggs are required.

1 cheese cup (Shredded)

1. 2. 3. 4. Directions:

5. 6. First and foremost, make sure you have all of the necessary fixings on hand. Whisk the eggs and yogurt thoroughly in a medium mixing bowl.

Add the cheddar, chives, ham, and pepper after that. Place your Instant Pot on a flat surface in your kitchen and turn it on.

This is a tremendous development. Open the lid and pour the mixture into the pot one at a time. Close the lid carefully and securely.

Close the valve as well later.

Press the "Slow Cook" button to begin making the recipe. Set the timer for around 85 to 90 minutes to allow for cooking.

Allow the blend to cook until the timer goes off in the pot.

There is one more task to do. Press "Drop" to turn off the pot. Allow the built-up pressure to naturally release; this will take 5 to 10 minutes.

Finally, the top of the container is opened. Serve warm wedges!

Time to prepare: 25–30 minutes

1 hour, 25 to 30 minutes of cooking time Serving Size: 2–3 A fondness for the past... Information about the calories:

There are 639 calories in a single serving of this recipe. 42.8 gram fat

9.5 grams of carbohydrate 1.9g of fiber

50.4 g of protein

Nut-Infused Super Oatmeal

To get your taste buds going, try these suggestions.
Ingredients:

almond flakes, 4 tblsp.

1 tsp cardamom (approximately 1 tsp)

pecans (1/4 cup)

oatmeal, 2 cups

1 teaspoon extract of vanilla

1 quart of liquid

brown sugar (approximately 3.5 tblsp.)

milk, 2 c.

1 cream cup

walnuts, 1/4 c.

Directions:

First and foremost, make sure you have all of the necessary fixings on hand. Combine the pecans and walnuts with a fork.

Now In the Instant Pot, combine the cereal, water, brown sugar, milk, cream, vanilla extract, and cardamom.

Cook for 5 to 10 minutes on "Porridge" in the Instant Pot.

There is one more task to do. Remove the oats from the Instant Pot and stir after that.

Finish by sprinkling the almond chips over the top and serving.

5 to 10 minutes of prep time 2 to 5 minutes in the oven 6–8 people It's best to keep it simple.

Information on the diet:

260 kcal

16.7 g dietary fiber

protein 22.71 carbs 6 Creamy Banana Breakfast Breads Yes, you heard right. I'd been waiting for this formula. Ingredients:

3 bananas in ripe condition (Chopped)

Syrup of maple (optional)

1 cup cheese from Philadelphia

pecans (1/4 cup) (Chopped)

eggs (three)

a half gallon of 2.5% milk

2 tbsp sugar, melted about 2.5 tbsp coconut oil

6 cubed slices of toast

1 tblsp cinnamon (ground)

Directions:

First and foremost, make sure you have all of the necessary fixings on hand. Make cubes out of the toast bread.

Place 1 layer of bread cubes in a baking dish oiled with a little coconut oil.

This is a tremendous development. Cover the bread layer with sliced bananas and Philadelphia cheese.

Make as many layers as you want by repeating the steps.

After that, strew cleaved walnuts over the layers.

Whisk the eggs with the sugar, cinnamon, milk, and vanilla in a medium or large bowl, if it's not too much trouble, and carefully pour the mixture over the layers.

In your instant pot, add 1 cup of water and the steaming rack. On the trivet, place the baking dish.

There is one more task to do. Set the timer for 30 to 35 minutes after you secure the top and select "Porridge."

When the timer goes off, quickly deliver the strain, remove the cover, and serve with maple syrup.

15–20 minutes of preparation time 30 to 35 minutes of cooking 6–7 portions Taste legend.

Data that feeds your soul: There are 61 calories in this recipe.
6 g protien

20 g fats 45 g carbs

Exceptional Cheese Quiche with a light flavor. Ingredients:

•\s•\s•\s•\s•\s•\s•\s•\s•

1. 2. 3. 4. 5. 6. 7. instructions

8. milk (1/2 cup)

cheese in a cup, ruined a teaspoon of salt (approximately)

green onions, slashed

1/8 tsp. black pepper, ground 4 bacon slices and cooked,
crumbled ham, diced

1 cup ground sausage (cooked)

6 massively beaten eggs all around

First and foremost, if it's not too much trouble, double-check
that you have all of the necessary ingredients on hand. Place
the trivet in the lower part of your Instant Pot and fill it halfway
with water.

Place the eggs, milk, salt, and pepper in a separate bowl at the
same time; then, whisk all of the ingredients together as one.

This is a tremendous development. Add the bacon, wiener, ham, green onions, and cheddar cheese until the soufflé dish is covered by about 1 quart.

Then, pour the egg mixture over the meat's highest point and thoroughly combine. In the Instant Pot, cover your soufflé dish and place your skillet on the trivet using aluminum foil.

Close the lid and set the timer for 30 to 35 minutes on high strain.

There is one more task to do. Turn off your Instant Pot and quickly release the pressure when the clock signals.

Finally, top the quiche with cheddar and cook until golden brown; then serve and enjoy!

30–35 minutes 3–4 portions As implied by the title.... Facts that are good for you: 139g fats 5g calories

40.0 milligrams of cholesterol

Carbohydrates in their Total Form 14g 9 g protien

Fruited Steel-Cut Breakfast Oats are fantastic...

Ingredients:

1 cup Greek yogurt, plain

slivered almonds (approximately 2.5 tblsp.) 1/2 gallon of water 2 peeled and cored apples 1 tsp

powder de cinnamon maple syrup, 1/4 cup

1 cup oats, steel-cut

1 teaspoon minced garlic

Directions:

First and foremost, make sure you have all of the necessary fixings on hand. In an Instant Pot, place the oats.

Add the water, yogurt, cloves, apples, maple syrup, and cinnamon and stir to combine.

Seal the valve by closing the cover.

Then press the Manual button and cook for 2 to 5 minutes according to the manufacturer's instructions.

There is one more task to do. Quickly release the strain.

Finally, re-mix and top with more maple syrup or cinnamon, as well as fragmented almonds.

2 to 4 servings

2–5 minutes of preparation time 5–10 minutes of cooking time You've got it. Data on nutrition:

Serving size: 330 calories

83.9 g carbs 10.4 g Protein 4.3 gram fat 12.1 g cellulose

Believe me when I say that this Strawberry Cream Oatmeal is a happy breakfast. Ingredients:

•\s•\s•\s•\s•

•\s•

Directions:

water, 1/4 cup

2 quarts strawberries (chopped) 8 quarts strawberries (chopped) milk, 1/4 cup

sugar, 1/4 cup

1 tsp sodium 2 cups oats that haven't seen the light of day

Cinnamon powder, 1/2 teaspoon

First and foremost, make sure you have all of the necessary fixings on hand. Then toss everything into the Instant Pot at the same time. Keep a few strawberry slices aside for garnish.

Secure the cooker's lid and select "Multigrain option" from the menu.

Allow 5 to 10 minutes for cooking.

There is one more task to do. Release the tension normally and remove the lid after the signal has been received.

Finally, slashed strawberries are placed on top.

4 to 6 servings

5 to 10 minutes of prep time 5–10 minutes of cooking time

I was always thinking about how it was put together... I finally got it one day while sitting next to my gourmet expert.

Data on nutrition:

There are 436 calories in a single serving of this recipe. 75 grams of carbohydrate 14.7 g Protein

8g fat 22 g Sugar

360 mg of sodium

Seafood & Fish

The best combination ever... Fantastic Creamy Coconut Fish Curry Are you not in agreement with me?

Ingredients:

2 c coconut cream

sour cream

curry powder (approximately 3.5 tblsp)

powder fenugreek seeds, ground

tomato

1 tblsp. chili powder (chopped)

a half teaspoon of powdered sugar

2 green chilies 1 tsp. turmeric (Sliced)

2.5 teaspoons finely ground

cumin 1 tbsp coriander seeds

Onions, medium (Sliced) 6 leaves of bay leaf

1.5 teaspoons grated fresh ginger two cloves of garlic

1 1/2 pound rinsed and cut-up fish fillets

Directions:

First and foremost, make sure you have all of the necessary fixings on hand. With a cooking splash, saturate the moment pot from the inside. Set the instant pot to the sauté setting.

Then, for about 2 minutes, add the garlic, ginger, and onion to the pot and sauté.

This is a tremendous development. Cook for 2 to 5 minutes after adding all of the ground flavors.

Stir in the coconut milk until it is thoroughly combined.

Tomatoes, fish, and green chilies are now added to the mix. Make a thorough mixture.

Cook on manual high strain for 5 to 10 minutes after tenderly sealing the pot with the cover.

Open the lid after releasing pressure with a quick delivery technique.

There is one more task to do. Add salt and pepper to taste.

Finally, stir everything together thoroughly before serving.

4 to 5 servings

10 to 15 minutes for preparation 15–20 minutes of cooking time This is something for which someone has unquestionably planned.

Information about the calories: 726 cals 50.8 grams total fat

30.4 grams of saturated fat 29.7 g Protein 46.8 g of carbs

7.1g fiber 7 g sucrose

Paella with Butter Shrimps is a fantastic dish.

Recipe is fantastic!!

Ingredients:

•\s•\s•\s•\s•\s•\s•\s•\s•\s•\s•\s•\s•

parsley, 1/4 cup Toss in some cilantro. 1 teaspoon of salt 2 cups broth de poulet 1 squeezed lemon

saffron, 1 tsp.

Garlic, 4 cloves (Chopped) shrimp (1 pound)

Fish fillet weighing about 1.5 pound As needed, red pepper 1 pound rice, long grain seasoning to taste

1 teaspoon of butter

1. Follow the steps below:

2.

3.

4.

5.

6.

7. 8.

9.

10. 11.

To begin, double-check that you have all of the necessary supplies. Place your Instant Pot on a flat surface in your kitchen and turn it on.

Open the top and add the shrimps, water, and fish to the pot one at a time.

Close the top of the box carefully and securely. Later, seal the valve as well. This is a tremendous development. Press the "Manual" button to start the formula.

Set the timer for around 5 to 10 minutes to begin cooking. Then, until the timer goes off, leave the saucepan to simmer the mixture.

Press "Cancel" to turn off the pot.

Allow the built-up pressure to naturally release; this will take 5 to 10 minutes. Toss in the spread, pepper, rice, and salt after opening the top.

Combine the red pepper, garlic, and lemon juice in a large mixing bowl and stir well. Add the "Manual" button in saffron. Then you must decide on a cooking time; set the timer at about the time the stock will be ready. Press 20 to 25 minutes with the lid closed.

There is one more task to do. Allow the mixture to simmer until the timer goes off in the cooker. Pressure is applied quickly.

Finally, top with cilantro and serve immediately.

5–10 minutes of preparation time 25–30 minutes of cooking time 8 to 10 lucky servings

Information about the calories: 397 kcal Fat\s23g 25.4 g carbs 2 g fibre

19 g protien

Chapter Three

Tomato-Sauced Calamari

This is, without a doubt, well-known!

Ingredients:

1 onion, blanched

lime juice (1 teaspoon)

1 tsp cilantro

3 cloves garlic

1 tsp white pepper powder

1 t. ginger powder

1/4 cup stock made from fish

1.5 tsp. thyme (fresh)

3 tomatoes, medium

1 quart of wine

water, 1/4 cup

Calamari (12 ounces)

1 teaspoon of extra virgin olive oil

Directions:

To begin, double-check that you have all of the necessary supplies. Carefully wash and remove the calamari.

The calamari should now be sliced into medium-thick pieces.

C. bounce the new herbs and tomatoes after slicing the garlic cloves and diceing the onion.

This is a tremendous development. Select "Sauté" mode on the Instant Pot.

Then, drizzle the olive oil over the sliced calamari in the Instant Pot. For 5 to 10 minutes, sauté the meal.

In a large Instant Pot, combine the garlic, thyme, onion, and tomatoes.

Sprinkle the water, ground ginger, wine, lime juice, and fish stock over the top of the dish, mix well, and cover.

There is one more task to do. Select "Meat/Stew" on the Instant Pot's menu. 5–10 minutes of simmering

Finally, remove the Instant Pot's cooked calamari. The meal should be served warm.

10 to 15 minutes of prep time 15–20 minutes of cooking time 4–6 people Wow, that's adorably adorable!!

Information about the calories: 238 calories, 6.1 grams of fat, 2 grams of fiber, 16.64 grams of carbohydrates, and 29 grams of protein

Shrimp with Spicy Cajun and Lime (Gluten-Free) Something new for a fresh start!!

Ingredients:

1 asparagus bundle, new

wedges made from lime

1 tablespoon Cajun seasoning - if it's not too much bother, double-check the contents.

fresh stripped shrimp, 1 pound

Directions:

First and foremost, make sure you have all of the necessary fixings on hand. In the Instant Pot, add 1 cup of cold water.

Place the steam rack in place and add the asparagus.

Place the shrimp on the asparagus with care and season to taste with Cajun.

One thing still needs to be finished. Then, at that point, secure the cover, select "Steam" and cook appropriately at low tension for around 2 minutes.

Finally when the time is up, fast delivery the strain and serve promptly and lime wedges.

Preparation time: 5 to 10 min Cooking time: 5 to 10 min Servings: 4 to 6 Try this my

way!!

Nutritional information: Calories: 126 Protein:

4.6 g Fats:

18g Carbs:

2.2g

Vintage Mussels In Citrus Juice And Dry White Wine

I don't be familiar with you, yet I incorporate this one everytime I get a chance.

Ingredients:

2 dozen cleaned mussels

To taste, a pinch of black pepper

cornmeal (1 cup)

Garlic cloves, about 2.5 (Minced)

1 teaspoon freshly squeezed lemon juice

salt (a pinch)

1 teaspoon freshly squeezed orange

5 c. water, chilled

parsley (about 2.5 tbsp) (Minced)

a third of a cup of white wine that is dry

1/2 pound prosciutto di Parma (Chopped)

olive oil (1/2 cup)

cilantro, minced (about 2.5 tbsp)

Directions:

First and foremost, make sure you have all of the necessary fixings on hand. In a mixing dish, combine cornmeal and mussels.

Pour cold water over the mussels and make sure they're completely immersed.

Allow for 1 hour of mussel dousing.

Ensure that mussels have been rinsed thoroughly after 60 minutes.

This is a tremendous development. Fill the Instant Pot Pressure Cooker with olive oil as you wait. "Saute" is pressed.

After that, cook for 2 to 5 minutes with garlic and Italian prosciutto. Using salt and pepper, season to taste.

Combine the orange and lemon juices, dry white wine, and mussels in a large mixing bowl.

Set the lid in place and lock it in place. Cook for 2 to 5 minutes with high tension.

Select the Quick Pressure Release option when the signal sounds.

There is one more task to do. For around 5 to 10 minutes, this will decompress. Remove the lid and throw it away.

Finally, sprinkle parsley and cilantro over top. Serve. 2 to 4 servings 1 1/2 CUP RECOMMENDED SERVING The secret is to bake!!

Data on nutrition: There are 146 calories in a single serving of this recipe. 0 gram of carbohydrate 4 gram of fat 20 gram protein

Fish Curry of the Year

I'm going to say it again... Assume you'll need it, and give it a go. Without hesitation. Right!! Ingredients:

•\s•\s•\s•\s•\s•\s•\s•\s•\s•\s•\s•\s•\s•\s•

1 piece of tomato (Chopped)

lemon juice (about 2.5 tblsp.) coconut milk, 14 ounces

1 tsp. cayenne 2 onions (sliced) 2 capsicums (cut into strips) Garlic cloves, about 2.5 (Minced) 6 curry leaves, powdered 1/2 teaspoon fenugreek

1 tbsp. ground coriander to taste with salt and black pepper 1 tsp. finely grated ginger

6 fish filets, chopped into medium pieces 1/2 teaspoon turmeric powder 2 tablespoons cumin powder

Directions:

First and foremost, make sure you have all of the necessary fixings on hand. Set

Set your moment pot to Sauté, add the oil and curry leaves, and cook for 2 minutes.

After that, add the ginger, onion, and garlic, combine well, and simmer for 2 to 5 minutes, depending on your preference.

Mix in the coriander, cumin, turmeric, fenugreek, and hot pepper, then simmer for 2 to 5 minutes, depending on how spicy you want it.

There is one more task to do. Add the coconut milk, tomatoes, fish, and capsicum now, stir to combine, cover, and simmer on Low for 5 to 10 minutes.

Finally, season to taste with salt and pepper, mix well, divide into bowls, and top with lemon juice. Enjoy!

10 to 15 minutes for preparation 15–20 minutes of cooking time 6–7 servings

Information about the calories:

230 calories, 10 grams of fat, 3 grams of fiber, 12 grams of carbohydrates, and 23 grams of protein

Sweet Soy Fish Reminiscences

Make your presence felt!! 3 tbsp. veg.

oil soy sauce, 3 tblsp

2.5 tblsp. garlic (minced) 2 tablespoons red chili, chopped 3 teaspoons shallot Galangal, 1 inch fresh trout (1 pound) Approximately 1 bay leaf

Directions:

To begin, double-check that you have all of the necessary supplies. Preheat the Instant Pot for 30 to 35 seconds, then choose the "Sauté" option from the menu.

Fill the Instant Pot with vegetable oil and brown the fish at this stage.

After removing the carmelized fish from the Instant Pot, put it aside.

This is a tremendous development. Return the sautéed fish to the Instant Pot after the oil has been disposed of.

Then top the fish with chopped garlic, shallots split in half, and red bean stew, followed by galangal and straight leaf.

Drizzle soy sauce over the fish, then fully cover the Instant Pot.

Select "Manual" and cook the spaghetti for 5 to 10 minutes on high.

There is one more task to do. Deliver the Instant Pot as soon as it's done, then open the cover.

After that, transfer to a serving plate and enjoy right away.

2 to 4 servings

5–10 minutes of preparation time 10–15 minutes of cooking time Add some zest to your life!

Information about the calories: 258 kcal 22 grams of fat

4.3 grams of saturated fat 10.7 g Protein 5 g of carbs

0.6g fiber 0.9g sugar

Snapper with a Spicy Kick So, what're your thoughts on the matter?

Ingredients:

•\s•\s•\s•\s•\s•\s•\s•\s•\s•\s•

1 (clean) red snapper A dash of salt from the sea

Bean stew paste (about 3.5 tablespoons) sesame oil, 1 tblsp.

1 tblsp soy

1 shallot (Chopped) 2 c.

Sesame seeds, roasted (about 2.5 tablespoons) a clove of garlic (Minced) sugar, 2 tsp

1 tsp. grated ginger

1. 2. 3. 4. 5. 6. 7. 8. 9. 10. 11. Directions: 1. 2. 3. 4. 5. 6. 7.

First and foremost, make sure you have all of the necessary fixings on hand. Cut a few slits in the snapper, season with salt, and set aside for about 25 to 30 minutes.

Place your Instant Pot on a flat place in the kitchen, plug it in, and turn it on.

Fill up the pot with water. Place the fish over the trivet and arrange the liner bin in the pot. The stew mixture should be rubbed on the snapper.

This is a tremendous development. Close the lid carefully and securely. Later, seal the valve as well.

Then hit the "Manual" button to start creating the formula. Set the timer for 10 to 15 minutes to start the cooking process.

Allow the mixture to simmer until the timer goes off in the cooker. Press "Cancel" to turn off the pot.

Allow the built-up pressure to naturally release; this will take around 5 to 10 minutes.

Open the lid and transfer the cooked mixture to the serving compartments.

There is one more task to do. Toss the sugar with the soy sauce, sesame seeds, garlic, ginger, sesame oil, and green onion in a medium-sized mixing bowl.

Finally, top the fish with the sauce you've prepared. 20 to 25 minutes of preparation time

10 to 15 minutes to cook

Serving Size: 2–3

What distinguishes this as the most effective? Take a look at it! Information about the calories:

186 calories, 12 grams of fat, 12 grams of carbohydrates 23.5g 1 g fibre 6.22 g protein

Marjoram Salmon in King Size

It's only gotten better! Ingredients:

•\s•\s•\s•\s•\s•\s•\s•\s•

marjoram, 1 tsp

1 tsp onion powder rosemary, half a teaspoon

1 tablespoon margarine

salt, 1 tsp dill, 1/2 cup

paprika (about 1.5 tbsp.) 1 quart of liquid

1 teaspoon cilantro 1 pound filet de saumon

Directions:

First and foremost, make sure you have all of the necessary fixings on hand. Fill a small bowl halfway with rosemary, marjoram, and salt.

Rub the zest mixture all over the salmon filet.

Now quickly cut the dill and combine it in a mixing bowl with the onion powder and paprika. Stir in the cilantro.

This is a tremendous development. Transfer the salmon filet to the Instant Pot's liner rack. Select "Steam" on the Instant Pot's menu.

The dill mixture should now be sprinkled over the fish.

Cook the fish for 15 to 20 minutes in the Instant Pot.

There is one more task to do. Release any remaining strain and allow the fish to rest momentarily after the cooking time has expired.

Transfer the dish to a serving platter at the last minute.

10 to 15 minutes of prep time 15–20 minutes of cooking time 6–7 portions I had a brilliant idea!!

Information about the calories: 127 calories, 6.2 grams of fat, 1 gram of fiber, 1.17 grams of carbohydrates, and 16 grams of protein

Salmon & Spinach Penne is a delicious combination of salmon and spinach. Enjoy this recipe as you relax!!

Ingredients:

1.5 tablespoons of extra virgin olive oil

to taste with pesto sauce

4 cup water that is still

to taste with salt and pepper

smoked salmon, 10 ounces, chopped into small pieces

1 pound of heavy cream

Lemon juice (about 1.5 tblsp)

16 ounces dry penne 1 cup parmesan cheese, grated

Directions:

To begin, double-check that you have all of the necessary supplies. In a large saucepan, combine the penne pasta, 4 cups water, and 1 tablespoon olive oil.

Close the lid, choose "Manual," and cook for 2 to 5 minutes at high tension.

Allow for a lengthy period for the tension to dissipate, and then quickly apply any remaining pressure.

Then, using a wooden spatula, carefully remove the top and stir in the smoked salmon chunks, heavy cream, lemon juice, 1/2 cup of parmesan, and spinach leaves.

There is one more task to do. Press "Saute" and heat until the leaves shrivel.

Finally, toss with the pesto sauce and the remaining 1/2 cup of parmesan.

10–15 minutes of preparation time 15 to 20 minutes to prepare 8- to 9-servings I had a brilliant idea!!

If you're up for a challenge, try this!! Information about nutrition: There are 420 calories in a single serving of this recipe. 13 g protien

11g fats 66 g carbs

Chicken & Poultry

What are your thoughts on this delectable chicken pot pie?

Ingredients:

Celery, 1/3 cup

1 tsp pepper (sliced)

a third of a cup of mixed frozen vegetables 1 cup broth made with chicken

1 tblsp chicken

seasoning dried thyme, about 1/2 tsp

Boneless and skinless chicken thighs, 10 oz onion, 1/4 cup (Chopped)

Directions:

First and foremost, make sure you have all of the necessary fixings on hand. Use the "Slow Cooker" setting on your Instant Pot if it's not too much trouble.

Now, quickly combine all of the ingredients in the slow cooker, excluding the frozen vegetables, and mix thoroughly.

Cook for 3 to 4 hours on low, covered.

There is one more task to do. Add frozen vegetables and cook for another 30 to 35 minutes on high.

Finally, enjoy your meal.

4 hours 40 minutes to 45 minutes total Time for a notable recipe. Serves: 2 to 3 Information about nutrition:

338 kcal

Carbohydrates: 11.3 g Fat 3.1 g protein, 10.5 g sugar 45.5 gram

126 milligrams of cholesterol

Magical flavor. Tasty Classic Spiced Chicken Breasts Ingredients:

•\s•\s•\s•\s•\s•\s•\s•

oregano, 1/8 tsp (Dried) 1 quart of liquid

1 tablespoon basil leaves, dried

Boneless and skinless chicken bosoms, 3 1 teaspoon of extra virgin olive oil

garlic powder, 1/4 teaspoon 1/4 teaspoon cayenne salt, 1/2 teaspoon

Directions:

First and foremost, make sure you have all of the necessary fixings on hand. Combine garlic powder, oregano, salt, dark pepper, and basil in a medium-sized blending bowl.

Now wash the chicken, pat dry, and spread 1/2 of the arranged mix on one side.

Place your Instant Pot on a flat surface in your kitchen and turn it on.

Press the "Sauté" button to begin making the formula.

This is a tremendous development. Cook for 2 to 5 minutes on each side to relax the ingredients, then add the oil and chicken, prepared side down.

Taking it out of the pot Fill up the pot with water.

Then, in the pot, arrange the trivet and place the chicken on top.

Close the top of the box carefully and securely. Later, seal the valve as well.

Press the "Manual" button to start the formula.

After that, set the timer for 5 to 10 minutes of cooking.

Allow the mixture to cook until the timer goes off on the clock.

Press "Cancel" to turn off the pot.

Allow the built-up pressure to naturally release; this will take around 5 to 10 minutes.

There is one more task to do. Open the lid and transfer the cooked mixture to the serving compartments.

Lastly, serve hot!

10 to 15 minutes of preparation time 15 to 20 minutes to cook 3–4 servings Vintage overabundance... Data on nutrition: There are 324 calories in a single serving of this recipe. 9.3 grams fat Carbohydrates\s19.5g 2 g fibre 42.3 g (protein)

The all-powerful Titanic Tomato Chicken Stew Ingredients:

sugar 1 tbsp

sweet potato (3 oz.)

1 pound boneless chicken breast with 1.5 teaspoon salt

oregano, 1 tblsp.

cilantro, 1 teaspoon

olive oil, 2 tablespoons

1.5 teaspoon ginger, freshly grated

carrots (two)

3 shallots

scallions (3 oz.)

shallots, 5 oz.

1 tsp dark pepper, ground

half-cup of heavy cream

Tomato juice (1/2 cup)

3 cup stock (chicken)

Directions:

To begin, double-check that you have all of the necessary supplies. In a blending bowl, whisk together the tomato juice, salt, cilantro, oregano, ground dark pepper, and cream.

The onions, yams, and carrots should now be stripped.

Make medium-sized pieces out of the vegetables.

This is a tremendous development. Select "Sauté" mode on the Instant Pot.

Sprinkle the olive oil over the hacked vegetables in the Instant Pot. Cook for 5–10 minutes, depending on the vegetables.

After that, stir in the tomato juice mixture. Shallots and scallions should be chopped finely.

Into the Instant Pot, add the slashed fixings.

Now, roughly chop the boneless chicken breast and place it in the Instant Pot, followed by the chicken stock.

Close the Instant Pot lid after stirring well with a spoon. 10. There is one more task to do. Cook for about 30 to 35 minutes on "Meat/Stew" mode.

11. Remove the stew from the Instant Pot and place it in serving bowls once it's finished cooking.

15 to 20 minutes of prep time 35–40 minutes of cooking time 8- to 9-servings For all of you, another fantastic formula... Information about the calories:

349 kcal

19.1 grams of fat

34.85 g of carbs

Salsa de Pollo de Pollo de Pollo de Pollo de Pollo de Pollo

For the most fantastic of people.

Ingredients:

•\s•\s•\s•\s•

Directions:

Salsa verde (16 oz.) smoked paprika (1 teaspoon) Cumin (approximately 1.5 tsp) 1 tblsp. sodium bicarbonate

Boneless chicken breasts, 2 1/2 pound

First and foremost, make sure you have all of the necessary fixings on hand. In your Instant Pot pressure cooker, combine all of the ingredients.

Select "Manual," then "High" pressure for 25 to 30 minutes.

When the timer beeps, the pressure is on for a quick delivery.

Chapter Four

Chicken Curry with a Kick

There is one more task to do. Shred the chicken carefully after opening the cooker.

Finally, enjoy your meal.

Prep + Cook Time: 25–30 minutes Servings: 6–8 This recipe is simple but tasty.

Information about the calories:

340 cals Fiber: 0 Fat: 7 Fat: 7 Fat: 7 Fat: 7 Fat: 7 Fat: 7 Fat: 7

6 oz. carbs

59 grams protein For you, we have a simple Orange Spice Chicken recipe... Ingredients:

•\s•\s•\s•\s•\s•\s•\s•\s•\s•

•

Directions:

2 tbsp. oil

orange zest and 4 green onions 2.5 heads of garlic (Minced) 1 quart sauce de tomato

to taste with salt and pepper 1 quart juice of orange

Soy sauce, 1/4 cup

corn starch (approximately 4.5 tblsp.) lb chicken bosom cut into two-inch pieces 1/4 cup granulated sugar brown sugar (1/4 cup)

First and foremost, make sure you have all of the necessary fixings on hand. Using a paper towel, pat dry the chicken.

In the cooker's pot, pour in the oil and chicken.

Cook the chicken for 2 to 5 minutes on medium-high heat, blending constantly, using the'sauté' key.

This is a tremendous development. Add the remaining fixings to the pot when the chicken has turned a brilliant brown color.

After that, thoroughly combine all of the components.

Close the cooker lid and secure it.

Set the timer for 5 to 10 minutes after selecting the 'poultry' option.

Use'regular delivery' to vent the steam for 10 to 15 minutes after the finish signal has been received. Then, and only then, should the lid be opened.

In a separate bowl, combine the cornstarch and the squeezed orange; add to the pot.

Then choose the 'sauté' function and cook the chicken for 5 to 10 minutes in the sauce.

There is one more task to do. Continue to stir until the sauce thickens.

Finish with cleaved green onions and a sprinkling of orange zing.

6 to 7 servings

15 to 20 minutes of prep time 15–20 minutes of cooking time Delightful... Data on nutrition:

818 cals 23.7 grams of carbohydrate 128.2 g protein

19.6 gram of fat 19.6g sugar

Sodium:

1120g

Like no other time, a wonderful chicken and potato dish...

Ingredients:

Skinless and boneless chicken thighs, 2 pound

to taste with salt and black pepper

1 quart chicken broth

lemon juice (1/4 cup)

Italian seasoning (approximately 2.5 tbsp.)

2 lb. red potatoes, quartered

olive oil, 2 tablespoons

Dijon mustard (approximately 3.5 tblsp.)

Directions:

First and foremost, make sure you have all of the necessary fixings on hand. Set your moment pot to sauté mode, add the oil, heat it up, add the chicken thighs, season with salt and pepper, mix well, and brown for 2 to 5 minutes.

There is one more task to do. Combine stock, mustard, Italian seasoning, and lemon juice in a mixing bowl; stir well. Pour over chicken, along with potatoes; cover and cook on High for 15 to 20 minutes.

Finally, serve by dividing the mixture among plates. Enjoy!

15 to 20 minutes for preparation 15–20 minutes of cooking time Worth it... Servings: 4–6

Information about the calories:

190 calories, 6 grams of fat, 3.3 grams of carbohydrates, and 18 grams of protein

Every now and then, my sister makes it. Ingredients:

tbsp flour + tbsp oil

2.5 teaspoons finely ground

coriander Tomatoes, 14 oz can (Chopped) garam masala, 2 tsp

turmeric (1 teaspoon)

2.5 tsp. 2 green chilies (chopped)

1 tsp ginger, ground cumin (Grated)

a couple of onions

1 lemon juice (chopped)

four crushed garlic cloves

4 boneless chicken thighs, diced

Directions:

To begin, double-check that you have all of the necessary ingredients. Now, set your Instant Pot to "Slow Cooker."

In a blender, combine the ginger, garlic, chilies, and onion until smooth.

Over medium heat, quickly heat the oil in the pan.

This is a critical step. Cook for 2 to 5 minutes after adding the blended puree to the pan.

After that, add the spices and cook for 2–5 minutes.

In a large mixing bowl, combine the flour and tomatoes.

Half-fill the tomato can with water and pour into the pan. Make a good stir.

Season the chicken with pepper and salt in the Instant Pot now.

Add lemon juice to the pan mixture and pour over the chicken. 10. There is still one thing to do. Cook for about 5 to 6 hours on low, covered.

11. Finally, serve and take pleasure in the meal.

6 hours 20 to 25 minutes total time

4 to 6 servings

To have an experience that will last forever.

Information about the calories:

387 kcal

Protein 44.9 g Cholesterol 130 mg Fat 14.8 g Carbohydrates 17.3 g Sugar 6 g

Thai Eggplant Chicken is fantastic. There are some things in life that will never let you down.

Ingredients:

•\s•\s•\s•\s•\s•\s•\s•\s•

6 chicken thighs, skinless and boneless, cut into small pieces
1 can coconut milk (approximately 1.5 tbsp)

red curry paste, 3 tblsp julienned basil leaves 2 tbsp sugar
Make halves out of 12 eggplants. chicken stock, 1/2 cup

2 tsp. soy sauce

1. 2. 3. 4. 5. 6. Directions:

7. Before you begin, double-check that you have all of the necessary ingredients. Place your Instant Pot on a flat area in your kitchen, plug it in, and turn it on.

Press the "Sauté" button to begin making the recipe. Cook for about 2 to 5 minutes to soften the ingredients, then add the curry paste, chicken, and 2 tablespoons coconut milk. This is a critical step. Add the fish sauce, eggplants, and the remaining coconut milk, as well as the stock. Then, with care, close and secure the lid. Seal the valve as well after that.

To begin, select "Manual" from the drop-down menu. Set the timer for 5 to 10 minutes to begin cooking.

Allow the mixture to cook until the timer goes off, then remove it from the pot. Press "Cancel" after turning off the pot. Allow the internal pressure to naturally release; this will take 5 to 10 minutes.

There is still one thing to do. Transfer the cooked mixture to serving container/containers after opening the lid. 11. Lastly, sprinkle basil leaves on top. Serve alongside rice or a salad of your choice.

5–10 minutes of preparation time

10 to 15 minutes to cook

Approximately 5–6 servings

Mushroom fries conjure up many memories for me. Information about the calories:

There are 388 calories in 388 calories in 388 calories in 388 calories in 388 calories 13 gram fat

55.2 grams of carbohydrates 25 g Fiber

13 grams of protein

Shredded Chicken is a dish that is known throughout the world.

You can do it in your spare time, sure... Ingredients:

sugar 1 tbsp

turmeric (1 teaspoon)

1 tsp. black pepper (ground)

1 tbsp. oil

3 cloves garlic

1 teaspoon salt 2 cups water 1 bay leaf

basil, 1 tsp

1 tsp butter

half-cup of heavy cream

1 lb. boneless chicken breast

Directions:

To begin, double-check that you have all of the necessary ingredients. Set the Instant Pot's pressure setting to "Pressure."

Fill the Instant Pot halfway with water and place the chicken breast on top.

The bay leaf should be added now. Cook for approximately 10 to 15 minutes with the lid closed.

This is a critical step. Release any remaining pressure and open the Instant Pot lid when the cooking time is finished.

Then, in a mixing bowl, shred the chicken breast.

Stir the sugar, ground black pepper, basil, salt, butter, cream, and turmeric into the shredded chicken until thoroughly combined.

Peel and finely mince the garlic cloves.

After spraying the inside of the Instant Pot with olive oil, add the shredded chicken.

There is still one thing to do. Cook for about 10 to 15 minutes on "Sauté" mode.

Transfer the dish to a serving plate once it's finished cooking. 10 to 15 minutes of prep time

20–25 minutes of cooking time

Supremacy defined!! Servings: 7 to 8 Information about the calories:

188 calories, 12 fat calories, and 1 gram of fiber

6.14 carbs

Excellent Italian Chicken Thighs (15 g protein)

My friends think I'm crazy for eating so much of this.

Ingredients:

2 medium carrots, peeled and chopped

To taste, season with salt

1 pound cremini mushrooms, stemmed and quartered

cherry tomatoes (about 2 cups)

3 garlic cloves, peeled and smashed

fresh Italian parsley, chopped

1.5 onion, finely chopped

1 tablespoon of extra virgin olive oil

1 cup fresh basil, thinly sliced

tomato paste (1 tbsp.)

1 tsp. black pepper (approximately)

8 chicken thighs (boneless, skinless)

Green olives, pitted, 1/2 cup

Directions:

To begin, double-check that you have all of the necessary ingredients. Sprinkle salt over the chicken thighs.

Now, press "Sauté" on your Instant Pot and add the olive oil.

Add the c mushrooms, carrots, onions, and a pinch of salt when the pan is shiny.

This is a critical step. Cook for 2 to 5 minutes, until the vegetables are soft.

Cook for 30 seconds more after adding the smashed garlic and tomato paste.

The cherry tomatoes, chicken thighs, and olives should be added last.

Before you lock the pressure cooker, turn off "Sauté."

Select "Manual" and "High" Pressure for 10 to 15 minutes.

There is still one thing to do. Quickly release the pressure when the beeper sounds.

Remove the lid and season with salt and pepper. Serve. 6–8 people

Time to prepare and cook: 25–30 minutes

So, how do you feel about it?

Information about the calories:

245 cals

3 g fibre

10 g carbs

35 Grain & Bean Protein

Kidney Beans (Boiled) Here's something new!!

Ingredients:

1 tsp sodium

1 c. white kidney beans (dried) 6 oz.

Directions:

To begin, double-check that you have all of the necessary ingredients. In the Instant Pot, combine all ingredients.

There is still one thing to do. The lid should then be closed and the vent should be sealed.

Finally, select Manual and set the timer for 40 to 45 minutes.

2 to 4 servings

2–5 minutes of preparation time 40–45 minutes of cooking time It will take some time and effort, but it will be worthwhile. Nutritional\sinformation: Serving Size: 56 Calories 3.4 g carbs 2.2 gram of protein

Fat:\s3.8g

Fiber:\s0.1g

Curry with Spinach and Chickpeas (Vintage Spinach & Chickpeas Prepare to do things the way I want!!

Ingredients:

1 1/2 tbsp. oil

fresh cilantro, chopped

1 pound onions, chopped

1 bay leaf, roughly 1.5 teaspoons salt (to taste)

1 garlic clove, grated

1/2 tsp ginger, grated

1 cup baby spinach, roughly chopped

water, 3/4 cup

1 quart pureed tomatoes

coarsely chopped 1/2 green chili

1.5 teaspoon cayenne pepper powder

Turmeric, 1/4 teaspoon

coriander powder, 1/2 teaspoon

chickpeas, raw

Directions:

To begin, double-check that you have all of the necessary items. In the Instant Pot, rapidly add the oil and onions. 5–10 minutes of "sautéing"

Now, combine the ginger, garlic paste, green chile, and bay leaf in a large mixing bowl. After 2 to 5 minutes of appropriate cooking, add all of the spices.

In a large saucepan, combine the chickpeas, tomato puree, and water.

This is a critical stage. Place the lid on top of the container and secure it. Set the pressure release handle to "seal."

Then cook for roughly 15 to 20 minutes on the "Manual" setting with high pressure.

Natural release for 20 to 25 minutes after the sound.

There is still one thing to do. On the "Sauté" setting, stir in the spinach and simmer for 2 to 5 minutes.

Finally, serve with a side of white rice that has been cooked.

4 to 5 servings

10 to 15 minutes of prep time 25–30 minutes of cooking time This is the most incredible combination!! Information about the calories:

180 kcal 25.3 grams of carbohydrate 6.7 gram of protein

7 g fat 6.9g sugar

Sodium is 79 milligrams per kilogram of body weight.

Risotto de Mushrooms Creamiest (Gluten-Free) Isn't it awesome?

Ingredients:

2 CUP PORTOBELLO MOUNTAINS (Sliced)

3 cups chicken broth 1/2 cup grated parmesan cheese

white wine (1/2 cup)

Approximately 1.5 onion (Diced)

1 tsp sodium chloride

two cloves of garlic

2 cups Arborio rice

2 tbsp unsalted butter – please check the ingredients

About 1.5 tbsp dried basil

Directions:

To begin, double-check that you have all of the necessary items. In your instant pot, melt 2 tablespoons unsalted butter by pressing the "Sauté" button, then sauté the onion and mushrooms for 2 to 5 minutes.

Add the Arborio rice and continue to cook for another 2 to 5 minutes, or until transparent.

Sprinkle with salt after carefully adding the white wine, chicken broth, and basil.

Then stir the rice with a wooden spoon, scraping the bottom to ensure no rice is trapped there.

There is still one thing to do. Secure the cover, press "Manual" on the pressure cooker, and cook for 5 to 10 minutes at high pressure.

Finally, after the timer goes off, immediately release the pressure, remove the cover, and top the risotto with grated parmesan cheese.

10–15 minutes of preparation time

10 to 15 minutes of cooking 6–7 portions

For you, a wonderful meal!! Information about the calories: There are 482 calories in a single serving of this recipe. Eleven grams of protein

15 g fats 48 g carbs

Porridge made with raw buckwheat. Simple yet brilliant!!

Ingredients:

•\s•\s•\s•\s•\s•\s•

Directions:

a cut banana Optional: sliced nuts

1 tblsp cinnamon powder vanilla extract (1/2 tsp.) rice milk (3 cups)

a quarter-cup raisins

a single cup groats of uncooked buckwheat To begin, double-check that you have all of the necessary items. Put the buckwheat in the Instant Pot after rinsing it.

The rice milk, banana, raisins, vanilla, and cinnamon are then added.

Make sure the valve is closed and the lid is shut.

This is a critical stage. Set the timer to around 5 to 10 minutes on "Manual," "High" pressure, and "Manual."

Unplug the pot and allow the pressure relax naturally for around 20 to 25 minutes after the timer whistles at the conclusion of the cooking cycle.

Stir in the porridge with a long-handled spoon.

There is still one thing to do. 4 bowls of porridge

Finally, to get the proper consistency, add extra milk to each serving. Sprinkle chopped nuts on top if desired.

Prep + Cook Time: 35–40 minutes Servings: 4–5

A new day has dawned.... Have you heard this one before?? Information about the calories:

247 cals

Carbohydrates: 54.3 Protein: 4.7 Fat: 2.6 Fiber: 4.4

Ham with Black-Eyed Peas This is a timeless classic.

Ingredients:

6 chicken stock (1/2 cup)

black-eyed peas, 1 pound dry ham, diced (5 oz.)

Directions:

Fill the Instant Pot halfway with water.

Seal the vent with the lid closed.

Change the cooking duration to 30 minutes by pressing the Manual button.

10 to 12 servings

2–5 minutes of preparation time 30–35 minutes of cooking time Now it's your turn to become a legend! Nutritional\sinformation: Serving Size: 90 Calories

9.1 g carbs 7.6 g protien 2.4 gram fat

Carrots, big ones

4.5 Season to taste with salt and pepper. 1 pound. beef (ground)

Directions:

First and foremost, make sure you have all of the necessary fixings on hand. Carrots should be sliced into 1/2-inch slices.

In a minute pot, combine the lumps and bone stock.

This is a tremendous development. Combine the beef, pepper, salt, garlic, and spinach in a medium or large mixing basin, and then shape into meatballs of appropriate size.

Then, on the carrot pieces, arrange the meatballs.

There is one more task to do. Close the lid and apply strong pressure for 15 to 20 minutes.

When the cooking is finished, release the tension and serve right away.

45 to 50 minutes total cooking time 4–5 portions

Try this one in the event that you're keen!! Information about nutrition: Calories: 192 Fat: 11g

Carbs: 3g Protein:\s32g

Sodium: 0.06g.

Great Garlic Spicy Sausage Meal Make me reminisce old fashioned days!!

Ingredients:

4 minced cloves

10 pieces of Italian Sausage

1 (15 ounces) can tomato sauce

1 (28 ounces) can chopped tomatoes

About 3 to 4 gigantic green bell peppers, grown, cored and form tiny bits

About 1.5 tablespoon basil

1 quart of liquid

About 1.5 teaspoons Italian seasoning

Directions:

First and foremost, make sure you have all of the necessary fixings on hand. Place your Instant Pot on a flat surface in your kitchen and turn it on.

Now open the top, and separately add the tomatoes, basil, pureed tomatoes, garlic powder,

In a saucepan, combine the Italian seasoning and water.

Do not mix in the frankfurter and pepper. Close the top of the box carefully and firmly.

This is a tremendous development. Later, seal the valve as well.

Chapter Five

Bacon-wrapped Collards

Nowadays, being healthy is a craze!! I keep speculating...

Ingredients:

•\s•\s•

•\sDirections:

1 tblsp. salt 1 pound collard greens, washed and stems trimmed black pepper, fresh ground

a quarter pound of bacon, sliced into 1-inch chunks

First and foremost, make sure you have all of the necessary fixings on hand. Spread the bacon on the bottom of the Instant Pot's internal pot right away.

Press the "Sauté" button and cook for 5 to 10 minutes, mixing occasionally, until the bacon is crisp and browned.

Cover a large tiny bunch of collard greens with bacon grease and cook until they are somewhat wilted. Add the remaining collards to the pot.

This is a tremendous development. Because they will quickly wilt, just pack them tightly enough to shut the top of the pot. After that, salt the greens and cover everything with water. The lid should be closed and locked.

Change the steam discharge valve to "Fixing," increase the strain to "High," and set the timer for 20 to 25 minutes.

Turn the steam valve to "Venting" to quickly release the tension when the clock goes off. Open the lid carefully and remove it.

There is one more task to do. Fill a serving dish halfway with collards.

Finally, freshly ground dark pepper is sprinkled on top, and then the dish is ready to be served.

6–7 servings Prep + cooking time: 40–45 minutes Wow!!

Information about the calories:

123 Calories

Carbohydrates: 4.4 Carbohydrates: 8.4 Fat: 8.4 Fat: 8.4 Fat: 8.4 Fat: 8.4 Fat: 8.4 Fat: 8.

Pinnacle Homemade Spaghetti Squash And Meat Sauce has a protein content of 8.7%.

Stunning and one-of-a-kind!!

Ingredients:

Onion

1 oz.

to use as a garnish cloves de usturoi 3 salt, kosher 1 and a half tablespoons

to flavor with black pepper

Squash spaghetti

Tomatoes, big (8 oz.)

Beef, ground1

1 pound of bay leaves

First, double-check that you have all of the necessary ingredients on hand. Add the onion, garlic, salt, and pepper to the meat in the saucepan.

Set the timer for 5 to 10 minutes in the cooker to sauté.

This is a tremendous development. Stir in the tomatoes, squished sound leaves, and cheddar.

Using a knife, pierce the spaghetti squash and place it over the sauce.

Then cover and simmer for 15 to 20 minutes, depending on the size of your pan.

There is one more task to do. Cut the spaghetti squash in half and scoop out the threads when it has cooled.

Serve the squash with the sauce and cheese on top.

30–35 minutes of total cooking time Iconic recipe of my rundown!! Servings: 5 to 7 Data that feeds your soul: 341 kcal 12g (fat)

17 g carbs 24 g protien 672mg of sodium

Eastern Lamb Stew is a show-stopping dish. It is, after all, a recipe from Grandma!! Ingredients:

1 sheep stew meat (1/2 - 13/4) pound

About 2.5 onions, diced 1/2 cup raisins (chopped)

a pound of garlic (Chopped)

salt, 2 tsp

chickpeas, rinsed and drained in 2 (15 oz.) jars

2 tsp cumin, 2 tsp pepper

coriander (about 2.5 tsp)

4 tablespoons honey or brown sugar, 2 1/2 cups chicken broth 2 teaspoons turmeric

cinnamon (two teaspoons)

1.5 teaspoon stew flakes (about)

4 TBS TOMATO POWDER

vinegar made with 1/2 cup apple juice

olive oil, 4 teaspoons

Directions:

First and foremost, make sure you have all of the necessary fixings on hand. On the current pot, choose the 'sauté' task.

Add the oil, garlic, and all of the seasonings now. 2–5 minutes of sautéing

Replace the cover and stir in all of the remaining ingredients.

Then, for 1 hour 15 to 20 minutes, switch the cooker to the 'meat stew' setting.

There is one more task to do. 'Normal delivery' the steam and remove the cover after the signal has been received.

Finally, add additional cilantro to the stew and serve.

8 to 9 servings

15 to 20 minutes of prep time

1 hour, 20 to 25 minutes of cooking time The time has finally come to be happy!! Data on nutrition: Calories:

87.2 g Carbohydrate, 65.4 g Protein, 44.2 g Fat

27.9g sugar 1018mg of sodium

When you're looking for a unique dish, try this charming Sausage Soup!! cups kale, kale leaves, kale leaves, kale leaves,

a half teaspoon of salt (chopped)

1 carrot 1 potato, diced (Grated) a quarter teaspoon of cayenne

1/4 cup heavy cream flakes flakes flakes flakes flakes flakes flakes

Italian sausage (1/2 pound),

2 3/4 cup chicken broth that has been browned

Directions:

To begin, double-check that you have all of the necessary supplies. Currently, please use your Instant Pot's "Slow Cooker" mode.

Then, in the slow cooker, combine all of the ingredients and thoroughly stir them together.

There is one more task to do. Cook for 3 to 4 hours on low, covered.

Finally, stir everything together well before serving.

4 hours total 10–15 min

2 to 3 servings

What's the situation like? There's only one way to find out...

Information about the calories:

682 kcal

Carbohydrates 45.3 g Sugar 5 g Fat 39.8% Fat 39.8% Fat 39.8% Fat 39.8% Fat 39.8% Fat 39.8% Fat 39.8% Fat 39.8%

Protein Cholesterol level: 34.9 g 116 mg

Corned beef that's just right They are something I could eat all day!!

Ingredients:

potatoes that are red in color

2 tablespoons cornstarch (for gravy) 1.5 garlic cloves (medium) Onion

1 jar of spices

4 cups beef stock

2 1/2 pounds corned beef brisket 1 cauliflower

Directions:

First and foremost, make sure you have all of the necessary fixings on hand. Put the meat in the instant pot, along with the potatoes, garlic, and onion, and cover with the stock.

The flavors should then be sprinkled over the entire arrangement. 3. Close the lid and set the timer to somewhere between 40 and 60 minutes.

Low pressure for 45 minutes

This is a tremendous development. Remove the cover and cool after cooking.

Cook for another 10 to 15 minutes, depending on the size of the cabbage.

Remove the meat but leave the drippings in place.

There is one more task to do. With the drippings, add 2 tbsp cornstarch.

Finally, stir everything together and cook until it starts to bubble. Reduce the heat and slowly thicken the sauce.

Time to cook: 55–60 minutes total 6–7 portions This one has a different meaning... Data on nutrition: 228 kcal 16g (fat)

3 g of carbs 16 g protien One gram of sodium

Pork Pinnacle Savory Instant Salsa Pinnacle Savory Instant Salsa Pinnacle Savory Instant Sals

Take a break from your daily routine and try something new. Nobody knows what you'll find, but we can all hope.

Ingredients:

•\s•\s•\s•\s•\s•

two cloves of garlic (minced) as needed with pepper and salt green salsa (1 cup)

1 pound pork (cut into small pieces) 1 teaspoon cumin powder 1 shallot (Diced)

1. 2. 3. 4. 5. 6. 7. 8. 9. 10. Directions: 1. 2. 3. 4.

11. First and foremost, make sure you have all of the necessary fixings on hand. Place your Instant Pot on a flat surface in your kitchen and turn it on.

Press the "Sauté" button to start making the formula. Cook for a couple of minutes to relax the ingredients before adding the pork, onion, and garlic.

This is a tremendous development. Cumin and salsa should be combined. Close the top of the box carefully and firmly. Later, seal the valve as well.

Then press the "Meat/Stew" button to start making the formula.

Set the timer for about 30 to 35 minutes of cooking time. Allow the mixture to cook until the timer goes off on the clock.

Turn off the stove and choose "Cancel."

Allow the built-up pressure to naturally release; this will take 5 to 10 minutes. There is one more task to do. Remove the lid and transfer the cooked mixture to serving holders or containers.

Finally, top with your favorite vegetables and serve warm over rice.

5–10 minutes of preparation time 30 to 35 minutes to cook

Serving Size: 4–5

Sure, with your extra energy, you can do it... Information about the calories:

There are 206 calories in a single serving of this recipe. 13 gram fat

16.2 g carbs 0 g Fibre

7.3 grams protein

Lamb Shanks with a Twist from Italy I want to know more! Ingredients:\s•\s•

•\s•\s•\s•\s•\s•\s•\s•\s•\s•\s•

Directions:

carrots, garlic cloves, peeled and chopped; slashed Italian parsley a single individual (14 oz.) tomatoes that have been cooked in a fire

1.5 onion, yellow (Diced) tomato paste (1 tbsp.)

celery (3 stems) (Diced) coconut oil (1 tblsp.)

balsamic vinegar, 1 tblsp.

1 teaspoon red pepper flakes, squashed 1 cup beef broth

pepper, 1/4 tsp salt (1/2 teaspoon)

Sheep shanks weighing 3 pound

To begin, double-check that you have all of the necessary supplies. Using pepper and salt, season the lamb legs.

Now press the Instant Pot's "Sauté" key and wait for it to heat up.

Heat up the coconut oil.

Cook the lamb legs for 5 to 10 minutes, or until all sides are seared, once the oil is hot. Put yourself on a plate.

This is a tremendous development. In a large mixing bowl, combine the onion, garlic, celery, and carrots.

Season to taste with salt and pepper.

Cook, stirring occasionally, until the onion is translucent, taking care not to eat the garlic.

Add the tomato glue and the fire-simmered tomatoes. To blend, stir everything together. Fill the pot with the lamb legs.

Add the balsamic vinegar and hamburger stock.

To turn off the sauté feature, press the"Drop" key.

The lid should then be covered and secured.

Set the clock for 45 to 50 minutes by pressing the"Manual" key and setting the strain to "High."

When the Instant Pot's timer beeps, release the tension naturally for 10-15 minutes or until the valve drops.

To deliver any remaining strain, turn the steam valve. The lid should be opened slowly and cautiously.

There is one more task to do. In a serving plate, place the lamb legs. Toss the shanks in the sauce and serve.

Finally, top with fresh parsley that has been slashed.

Preparation + Cooking Time: 1 hour 10 to 15 minutes Servings: 4 to 5 Days that are wonderful!!

Information about the calories:

405 Calories

28.8 g fat

Carbohydrates: 13.3 Carbohydrates: 3.4 Fiber: 3.4 Fiber: 3.4 Fiber: 3.4 Fiber:

98.3 % protein

Korean Beef, King Size That is truly remarkable!!

1 pound lean beef, 1 pound green onion, 1 clove garlic, sliced

1 head of garlic Brown

14 cup sugar 1 tbsp. red pepper

Sesame oil2 tbsp. sodium soy sauce1/4 cup 1/2 teaspoon grated ginger

Directions:

To begin, double-check that you have all of the necessary items. Set the temperature of the moment pot to sauté and drizzle in the sesame oil.

Cook for 45 to 50 minutes after adding the hamburger with garlic.

Combine the ground ginger, soy sauce, red pepper flakes, and sugar in a mixing bowl. Make a great connection.

There is one more task to do. Close the cover immediately after that and set the timer for 5 to 10 minutes at high pressure.

Finally, after the tension has been released, serve the dish immediately.

45 to 50 minutes total cooking time 4–6 people

Is it possible for you to succeed? Why not, I say. Information about the calories: There are 280 calories in a single serving of this recipe. 13g (fat)

15 g carbs 23 grams of protein Sodium:

0.6g

The life of a legend begins with this Mighty Garlic Beef Sirloin.

Garlic powder, about 4.5 teaspoons

to taste with salt and pepper

8 garlic cloves (chopped)

Top sirloin steak from a 6 pound hamburger

1 tablespoon of butter

Directions:

To begin, double-check that you have all of the necessary supplies. On the current pot, choose the'sauté' task.

Then add the sirloin steaks and the oil.

This is a tremendous development. Cook for 5 to 10 minutes, depending on the recipe. Allow both sides of the meat to brown.

Remove the lid and stir in all of the remaining fixings.

Then switch to the'meat stew' setting on the cooker and cook for 30 to 35 minutes.

There is one more task to do. After the blare, remove the lid and 'normally deliver' the steam.

Last but not least, serve immediately.

8 to 9 servings

10 to 15 minutes of prep time 50–55 minutes of cooking time It's amusing and delicious!!

Information on health:

865 cals Carbohydrate:\s2g Protein:\s103.9g Fat:\s44.3g

0.4g sugar

368 g sodium

Pineapple Pork with a Twist

Something is clearly out of the ordinary.

fish tsp

sauce 1 tbsp sodium bicarbonate 1.5 teaspoons of extra virgin olive oil

pineapple, 1/2 cup (Diced)

1 pound pork shoulder, cut into two pieces with 1.5 teaspoon liquid smoke water (1/2 cup)

Directions:

To begin, double-check that you have all of the necessary supplies. In the moment pot, pour in the olive oil and choose the sauté option.

Burn the pork for 2 to 5 minutes on each side, or until it is lightly browned.

This is a tremendous development. Using salt, season pork.

In a large pot, combine the pork, fish sauce, pineapple, fluid smoke, and water.

Then cover the pot with the lid and cook for 85 to 90 minutes on the manual setting.

Open the lid after allowing normal delivery pressure.

There is one more task to do. Remove the pork from the skillet and shred it with forks.

Finally, enjoy your meal.

8 to 9 servings

10 to 15 minutes for preparation 90-95 minutes of cooking time This is absolutely incredible. Consider it!!

Information about the calories:

342 kcal 24.9 grams total fat

9 grams of saturated fat 26.5 g Protein 1.4 g carbs 0.1 g fiber

1.1g sugar

Tasty Berry Sauce In Minutes, Meatless Cuisines, Ketogenic, Main Dish Wow!! Wow!! Wow!! Wow!! Wow!! Wow!! Wow!! Wow!! Wow!!! Wow

Ingredients:

2 cups blueberries, plus a few extra for decoration

For garnish, 1/2 cup freshly toasted disintegrated pecans

2 cups raspberries, plus a few extra for decoration

1 quart of liquid

For garnish, use 1/2 cup dried coconut shavings

brown sugar (1/2 cup)

1 teaspoon freshly squeezed lemon juice

1 lengthwise split vanilla bean

2 cups strawberries, plus a few extras for decoration

Directions:

First and foremost, make sure you have all of the necessary fixings on hand. Fill the Instant Pot Pressure Cooker halfway with strawberries, blueberries, water, raspberries, earthy colored sugar, and a vanilla bean.

Now it's time to secure the top configuration. Cook for 10 to 15 minutes, depending on how hard you press the high strain.

This is a tremendous development. Select Quick Pressure Release when the blare sounds.

For around 5 to 10 minutes, this will decompress. Remove the lid and throw it away.

The spent vanilla bean should then be disposed of. Lemon juice should be added now.

Make adjustments to the recipe to suit your preferences.

Fill a submersion blender halfway with water and blend until smooth. Blend until the mixture is completely smooth. Chill.

There is one more task to do. Pour chilled natural product sauce over fresh berries before serving.

Finally, add disintegrated pecans and coconut shavings for a finishing touch.

1/4 cup is the recommended serving size. Data on nutrition: Carbohydrates - 5.4 grams - 20.6 calories 0 gram of fat

0.3 grammes protein

Green And Red Cabbage Braised

Corned Beef is a tasty dish to prepare. This one is for those who aren't afraid to break the mold. Ingredients:

•\s•\s•\s•\s•\s•\s•\s•\s•\s•

2 oz (Sliced)

water, 17 oz.

Garlic cloves, about 2.5 (Minced) to taste with salt and black pepper 11 ounces celery, thinly sliced 2 yellow onions

4 halved cinnamon sticks Dried dill (approximately 1.5 tblsp.)

meat brisket pounding with inlet leaves

Directions:

To begin, double-check that you have all of the necessary supplies. Place the hamburger in a bowl with enough water to cover it, set aside for a few hours to soak, then channel and transfer to your moment pot.

Then toss in the celery, orange slices, sound leaves, onions, garlic, dill, cinnamon, pepper, dill, salt, and 17 ounces of water.

There is one more task to do. Cook on High for 45 to 50 minutes, stirring occasionally.

Finally, transfer the meat to a cutting board, slice it, divide it among plates, and serve with the juices and vegetables from the pot. Enjoy!

10 to 15 minutes for preparation

60–65 minutes of cooking time 5–6 people Be surprised if I say so myself.

Information about the calories:

251 kcal

3.14 grams of fat, 0 grams of fiber, 0 grams of carbohydrates, 1 gram of protein

Cooking level is endless with this Mustard Spinach Instant Meal....

Ingredients:

•\s•\s•\s•\s•\s•\s•\s•\s•\s•\s•\s•\s•

ginger, 1" handle (Minced) fenugreek leaves, dried 2 c. diced onions Garam masala, about 1.5 teaspoon cumin 1 tsp

1 pound washed and dried spinach 1 tsp cilantro

a quarter teaspoon of black pepper mustard leaves, rinsed, about 1 teaspoon cayenne 1 tsp turmeric, 1 tsp salt

4 garlic cloves, 2 tablespoons ghee (Minced)

First and foremost, double-check that you have all of the necessary ingredients on hand. Place your Instant Pot on a flat surface in your kitchen and turn it on.

Press the "Sauté" button to start making the formula. \ Cook for 2 to 5 minutes to relax the ingredients with the ghee, garlic, flavors, and onions.

Cook until the spinach has wilted.

This is a tremendous development. Add the mustard greens now, then carefully close and lock the lid. Later, seal the valve as well.

Press the "Manual" button to begin creating the formula. You must now set the timer for 15 to 20 minutes of cooking.

Allow the mixture to cook until the timer goes off on the clock.

Press "Cancel" to turn off the pot.

Allow the built-up pressure to naturally release; this will take around 5 to 10 minutes.

There is one more task to do. Open the lid and transfer the cooked mixture to the serving compartments.

Last but not least, serve with warm bread!

5–10 minutes of preparation time 15 to 20 minutes to cook 5 to 6 servings uber delicious!!

Information about the calories: 80 Calories, 5g Carbohydrates, 80 Calories, 80 Fat Calories, 80 Calories, 80 Cal 6g 3 g fibre 4 grams of protein

Ingredients:

1 1/2 pounds red cabbage, sliced

1/2 tsp. salt 1 cup water

1 tablespoon of mushroom stock

Coconut oil (2.5 tbsp)

1 pound grated carrots

1/8 tsp sesame oil, toasted

red pepper flakes (1/2 teaspoon)

14 cup vinegar from coconut

a quarter cup of torn parsley tops

Brown sugar (approximately 1.5 tbsp.)

2 pound wedges of green cabbage

cayenne powder (about 1 tsp.)

slurry of cornstarch

Approximately 2.5 tsp cornstarch dissolved in...

water, 2 tbsp.

Directions:

To begin, double-check that you have all of the necessary supplies. Select "saute" from the drop-down menu. Fill the Instant Pot Pressure Cooker with extra virgin olive oil.

Cook the cabbage wedges for a few minutes, or until they're almost done.

Place on a plate to keep warm.

This is a tremendous development. Continue in the same manner until all of the cabbages are cooked.

In the crockpot, combine mushroom stock, red pepper drops, carrots, coconut vinegar, earthy colored sugar, and cayenne powder.

The top setup should be locked. Cook for 5 to 10 minutes, depending on how hard you press the high strain.

Select the Quick Pressure Release option when the signal sounds.

For around 5 to 10 minutes, this will decompress.

Take the cover off the table. Arrange the vegetables on a serving platter in a pleasing manner. Press the "saute" button for the sauce.

11. Finally, add the cornstarch slurry to the mixture. Cook, stirring occasionally, until the sauce has thickened. 12. Add salt and sesame oil. Alter the cooking method to suit your preferences.

There is one more task to do. To serve, arrange cooked vegetables on plates in an even proportion. Serve the vegetables with a sauce on top.

Finally, fresh parsley should be used to finish off the look.

4 to 6 servings

1 1/2 cup (approximately) Approach is long...

Data on nutrition: Carbohydrates (108 calories) 14:24 g 5.07 gms of fat

1.77 grams (protein)

Beef Bourguignon is a classic dish that has been around for a long time. It is critical to move quickly...

Ingredients:

•

•\s•\s•\s•\s•\s•\s•\s•\s•\s•

carrots (two) (Sliced)

to taste with salt and black pepper 1/2 gallon of beef stock

1 cup red wine, preferably dry

dried basil, about 1/2 teaspoon three cuts of bacon (Chopped)

cut into quarters 8 ounces mushrooms two cloves of garlic (Minced)

white flour (approximately 2.5 tbsp.) 12 onions, pearl

Round steak, 10 pounds, cubed

Directions:

First and foremost, make sure you have all of the necessary fixings on hand. Set your instant pot to Sauté mode and cook for 2 minutes with bacon and an earthy color.

Then add the meat and flour and cook for 5 to 10 minutes, stirring occasionally.

There is one more task to do. Mix in the salt, pepper, wine, stock, onions, garlic, and basil, cover, and cook for 20 minutes on High.

Finally, add the mushrooms and carrots, cover the pot again, and cook for another 5 to 10 minutes on High. Divide the mixture between plates and serve. Enjoy!

15 to 20 minutes for preparation 30–35 minutes of cooking time 6–8 people Make an excellent impression.

Information about the calories:

442 kcal

17.2 grams of fat, 3 grams of fiber, 16 grams of carbohydrates, and 39 grams of protein

Cauliflower Cauliflower Sweet Potato It's undeniably better to be fortunate.

Ingredients:

1 diced tomato (15 oz.)

1 peeled and chopped onion

nut butter (approximately 1.5 tblsp.)

cayenne pepper, 1/4 teaspoon

cumin seeds (1/2 teaspoon)

1 tsp sodium

1 washed and drained 15-ounce can chickpeas

3-garlic cloves

1.5 tbsp curry powder (distributed)

1 pound yams, peeled and cubed 1 large cauliflower head, peeled and cut into flowerets

1/8 teaspoon cinnamon 4 cups vegetable stock

cultivated and minced 1 small stew pepper

1.5 tsp ginger powder

3–4 c.

Directions:

To begin, double-check that you have all of the necessary supplies. Place your Instant Pot on a flat surface in your kitchen and turn it on.

Press the "Sauté" button to start making the formula.

Cook for 2 to 5 minutes to mellow the ingredients, adding the oil and onions as needed.

Cook for 30 to 40 seconds, stirring occasionally, until the cumin seeds, garlic, bean stew pepper, and ginger are fragrant.

This is a tremendous development. Close and securely lock the container after adding the cinnamon, stock, potatoes, and 1 teaspoon curry powder.

Close the valve as well later.

Press the "Manual" button to start the formula.

Set the timer for 2 to 5 minutes to start the cooking process.

Then, until the timer goes off, leave the pot to cook the mixture as directed.

Press "Drop" to turn off the pot. Allow the built-up pressure to naturally release; this will take 5 to 10 minutes.

Open the lid and press the "Sauté" button.

There is one more task to do. Just cook the cauliflower, 3 cups water, chickpeas, tomatoes, cayenne pepper, 2 teaspoons curry powder, and salt until the cauliflower is tender.

Finally, add the peanut butter and serve while it's still hot!

5–10 minutes of preparation time 10 to 15 minutes to cook Approximately 7 to 8 servings The plot thickens!!

Calories rotein - 18g Nutritional Information

Tomato Soup with Great Zucchini Noodles Recipe for a hit list

Ingredients:

Zucchini:

salt (a pinch)

Using a spiralizer, spiralize 4 zucchini into dainty strips.

dark pepper, a pinch

Soup

1 onion (1 cup)

For garnish, roughly 1/4 cup cleaved level leaf parsley

Garlic, grated (about 2.5 tbsp.)

1 tsp. paprika powder (sweet)

1 tsp. flakes de pimentón

1 tomato crate

1 cup olives (green, pitted)

1 c. julienned kale leaves

thyme powder (about 1/2 tsp.)

salt (a pinch)

red wine, 1/2 cup

3 cups vegetable stock a pinch of dark pepper

2 tablespoons of extra virgin olive oil

Directions:

To begin, double-check that you have all of the necessary supplies. Fill a colander halfway with zucchini noodles, salt, and pepper. Drain the contents.

Fill the Instant Pot Pressure Cooker halfway with olive oil to make the stew. "Saute" is pressed.

2 to 5 minutes, or until limp and translucent, sauté garlic and onion.

This is a tremendous development. Tomatoes, olives, vegetable stock, thyme powder, red wine, sweet paprika powder, and red pepper flakes are among the ingredients to use.

Salt & pepper to taste.

Set the lid in place and lock it in place. Cook for approximately 5 to 10 minutes on the manual setting.

Select Natural Pressure Release when the beep goes off. It'll take 20 to 25 minutes to decompress.

Take the cover off now. The machine should be turned off. Add kale leaves and toss to combine.

There is one more task to do. Place a portion of zoodles on a plate and serve.

Pour the stew on top at the end. Sprinkle parsley on top.

3 to 4 servings 3/4 cup recommended serving size Data on nutrition:

Carbohydrates: 11.5 grams Calories: 93.8 4.8 gram of fat

2.2 grams protein

Delicious Sauce And Happy Chicken

Mushroom fries conjure up many memories for me.
Ingredients:

•\s•\s•\s•\s•\s•

1.5% lemon juice cup Greek yogurt a pinch of salt and pepper

Grated ginger, about 1/2 teaspoon 1 tablespoon skinless, boneless, and chopped garam masala chicken bosoms

Sauce ingredients:

•\s•\s•\s•\s•\s•

4 finely minced garlic cloves cayenne pepper (approximately 1/2 tsp.)

15 oz. tomato sauce (in a can) turmeric powder (1/2 teaspoon)

paprika (approximately 1 tblsp.) garam masala, 4 tblsp.

Directions:

To begin, double-check that you have all of the necessary items. Blend the chicken with the lemon juice, yogurt, ginger, 1 tablespoon garam masala, salt, and pepper in a mixing bowl, then set aside for 1 hour in the ice chest.

Set your instant pot to sauté mode, then add the chicken, mix well, and cook for 5 to 10 minutes.

There is one more task to do. Then add 4 teaspoons garam masala, pureed tomatoes, garlic, paprika, turmeric, and cayenne, mix well, cover, and cook for 10 to 15 minutes on High.

Finally, divide the mixture evenly among the plates and serve. Enjoy!

1 hour, 10 to 15 minutes of preparation time 20–25 minutes of cooking time

4–6 people

Every now and then, my sister makes it. Calories 452, Fat 4, Fiber 7, Calories 452, Fat 4, Fiber 7, Total Calories 452, Total Calories 452, Total Calo

9

Chickpeas, Broccoli, and Protein 12 In order to have an experience that will last a lifetime. Ingredients:

•\s•\s•\s•\s•\s•\s•\s•

1 can chickpeas, drained (15 ounces) 1 teaspoon of extra virgin olive oil

if needed, crushed red pepper 3 gigantic garlic cloves fennel seeds (about a quarter teaspoon) 1 halved package of broccoli rabe

As needed, season

14 cup broth

1. 2. 3. Directions

To begin, double-check that you have all of the necessary supplies. Place your Instant Pot on a flat surface in your kitchen and turn it on.

Press the "Sauté" button to start making the formula. Cook for 2 to 5 minutes, until the garlic is golden brown.

This is a tremendous development. Cook for approximately 30 to 35 seconds after adding the seeds and red pepper.

The stock, broccoli, and chickpeas are then added.

Then, with care, close and secure its cover. Later, seal the valve as well.

Press the "Manual" button to start the formula.

Set the timer for 2 to 5 minutes to start the cooking process.

Allow the pot to cook the combination appropriately until the clock goes off.

Now switch off the pot and press"Cancel."

Allow the built-up pressure to naturally release; this will take 5 to 10 minutes.

There is one more task to do. Remove the lid and transfer the cooked mixture to serving holders or containers.

Lastly, serve hot! 5–10 minutes of preparation time

10 to 15 minutes to cook

3–4 servings Data on nutrition: Calories 506

10 grams fat 44.3 grams of carbohydrates 12 g cellulose

24.3 g (protein)

Limit This Dish To Once A Week Worth It...

1 pound al dente elbow macaroni

1 1/2 cups chicken thigh fillets

11/2 cups vegetable stock

salt (a pinch)

For the dressing

1 cup mayonnaise

Pinch of white pepper

3/4 cup raisins

1/2 cup celery, minced

3/4 cup carrots, grated

1 can smashed pineapple, drained

Directions:

To begin, double-check that you have all of the necessary supplies. For the chicken, put chicken filets, vegetable stock, and salt into the Instant Pot Pressure Cooker.

Now lock the cover put up. Press the high tension and cook correctly for roughly 25 to 30 minutes

This is a tremendous development. At the instant when the blare sounds, Choose the Quick Pressure

Release.

For around 5 to 10 minutes, this will decompress.

Then remove the top. The machine should be turned off.

Shred chicken. Set up pasta, chicken, and cooking fluid in a bowl.

To prepare the dish of mixed greens, top chicken spaghetti blend in with celery, pineapple, carrots, mayonnaise, raisins, and pepper.

There is one more task to do. Change preparation as suggested by your chosen flavor.

Finally cover with saran wrap. Place inside the fridge for approximately 1.5 hour or until ready to serve.

2 to 4 servings

Recommended Serving Size: 1 cup salad - limit this Nutritional data: Calories - 438.8\sCarbohydrates - 30.2 grams Fat - 22.6 grams Protein - 11.3

Simple formula for you...

Best Green Olives Instant Potatoes\sFor people who're incredibly terrific.

Ingredients:

1 1/2 cup diced carrots

4 cups potatoes, create reduced down pieces

2 c.

1 cup green peas

1 cup corn kernel

Make dressing:

1/4 cup + 1 tablespoon mayo

1 tsp sodium

1/2 teaspoon ground dark pepper

10 green olives, minced

Directions:

To begin, double-check that you have all of the necessary supplies. Place your Instant Pot on a flat surface in your kitchen and turn it on.

Now open the top, and separately place the carrots, potatoes, and water in the pot.

Close the top of the box carefully and securely.

This is a tremendous development. Later, seal the valve as well.

To begin creating the formula, hit "Manual" button. Presently you need to establish cooking time; set the clock for roughly 10 to 15 minutes.

Then, until the timer goes off, leave the saucepan to simmer the mixture.

Press "Cancel" to turn off the pot.

Allow the built-up pressure to naturally release; this will take 5 to 10 minutes.

Now open its lid and shift the mixture to a separate dish.

In the unfilled pot, add the corn and peas; seal the lid. Press"Manual" button.

You need to set cooking time; set the clock for roughly 2 minutes.

There is one more task to do. Move the cooked combo into serving compartment/containers.

Finally combine the dressing ingredients and potato combination, and blend thoroughly. Serve warm!

5–10 minutes of preparation time 15 to 20 minutes to cook Number of Servings: 6 to 7 Simple yet\sscrumptious dish.

Information about the calories: Calories 295 Fat\s9g Carbohydrates 45.2g Fiber - 6g Protein - 6.3g

Nostalgic Different Lasagna\sWizard of all recipes. Ingredients:

•\s•\s•\s•\s•\s•\s•\s•

8 ounces sliced mozzarella 1 pound ground meat

1.5 onion, yellow (Chopped) 20 ounces keto marinara sauce 1 egg 1 1/2 cup grated parmesan cheddar cheese 1 1/2 cup ricotta cheese minced garlic cloves (about 2.5 cloves)

Directions:

To begin, double-check that you have all of the necessary supplies. Set your instant pot to sauté, then add the onion, garlic, and beef, mix well, and cook for 5 to 10 minutes.

Now add the marinara sauce, stir well, and transfer half of the mixture to a bowl. In a separate dish, mix together the ricotta, parmesan, and egg.

This is a tremendous development. Half of the cheese should be spread in your moment pot.

After that, spread half of the ricotta mixture.

Toss in the remaining hamburger and marinara mixture, as well as the remaining mozzarella and ricotta mixture.

There is one more task to do. Cover the saucepan with tin foil and simmer for 10 to 15 minutes on high.

Finally, slice the lasagna and divide it among plates. Enjoy!

10 to 15 minutes for preparation 25–30 minutes of cooking time

8- to 9-servings

For all of you, another fantastic recipe... Information about the calories:

339 calories 339 calories fat 4 calories calories fat 4 calories calories fat 4 calories calories fat 4 calories

2 dietary fiber

Mighty Walnut Beet Lunch Bowl - 8 Carbs, 36 Protein

Ingredients:

•\sDressing:

2 cups water • 1 1/2 pounds scrubbed and washed beets

1 tsp mustard dijon

as required with pepper and salt

2.5 tsp apple cider vinegar

extra virgin olive oil, 1 1/2 teaspoons

sugar, 1 1/2 teaspoons

lemon juice (about 2.5 tsp)

pecans (2 tblsp) (Chopped)

Directions:

First and foremost, make sure you have all of the necessary fixings on hand. Place your Instant Pot on a flat surface in your kitchen and turn it on.

Open the lid and pour the water and beets into the pot one at a time. Close the lid carefully and securely.

Seal the valve as well afterwards.

Press the "Manual" button to start the formula.

This is a tremendous development. You must now set the timer for 10 to 15 minutes of cooking.

Then, until the timer goes off, leave the saucepan to simmer the mixture.

Press "Cancel" to turn off the pot.

Allow the built-up pressure to naturally release; this will take 5 to 10 minutes.

Open the lid and transfer the cooked mixture to a mixing basin.

Drain and chop the beets into smaller pieces. 11. In a blender, combine all of the dressing ingredients except the oil and walnuts in a mixing dish.

There is one more task to do. Slowly incorporate the olive oil into the dressing, ensuring that it is well included.

Finally, toss the beets with the dressing and serve!

5–10 minutes of preparation time 2–5 minutes of cooking time 2–3 servings Vintage overburden... Data on nutrition: 151 kcal

10 grams fat

15.2 grams of carbohydrates 3 g fibre 2.7 grams protein